101 Juice Diet Recipes

Juice Diet Recipes That Help You to Lose Weight, Boost Energy, Increase Immunity and Detox Body

Sarah Sparrow

PUBLISHED BY:

Sarah Sparrow

Disclaimer

The information contained in this book is for general information purposes only. The information is provided by the authors and while we endeavor to keep the information up to date and correct, we make no representations or warranties of any kind, express or implied, about the completeness, accuracy, reliability, suitability or availability with respect to the book or the information, products, services, or related graphics contained in the book for any purpose. Any reliance you place on such information is therefore strictly at your own risk.

Table of Contents

101 Juice Diet Recipes

Aromatic Juice Drink

This juice is loaded with vitamins and minerals that are good for the heart; help reduce blood cholesterol, and lower blood pressure. Rich in vitamin C and B-complex that helps the body develop immune resistance, improve the intestinal motility and has anti-inflammatory, painkiller, nerve soothing, anti-pyretic as well as anti-bacterial properties, this is a refreshing and aromatic juice drink.

1 cucumber
1 mango
2 stalk fennel with leaves
1 sprigs of mint
1/2 inch piece of ginger

Push all through juicer.

Note: mint leaves can be rolled up into a ball to create volume when pushing through the juice extractor. Stir and enjoy!

Celery Cucumber Cooler

Celery and cucumber are low-calorie vegetables but rich sources of dietary fiber, an ideal combination for weight loss. This is a refreshing mix of fruits and vegetables which are all rich in vitamins and anti-oxidants. This cooler can help reduce inflammation and give protection against cancer.

3 stalk celery
½ medium cucumber, peeled
2 apple, sliced
5 medium carrots, greens removed
1 lemon, sliced

Combine all ingredients together in the juicer, stir and serve.

Healing Juice

If you are suffering from high blood pressure, having blurry vision and heart problems, this is a healing juice for you. Vegetables are a rich source of vitamins and anti-oxidants to cure various health problems.

4-5 medium carrots

100g fresh spinach

100g leaf parsley

4-5 sticks of celery

Combine all ingredients together in the juicer. Stir and serve.

Mediterranean Juice

This is a recommended drink for those suffering from anemia since these vegetables are a rich source of iron along with other vitamins and minerals.

100g parsley

1-2 red pepper

1-2 cups broccoli florets

4 medium carrots

Put ingredients through juicer in the same order as the list. Add flavor in the mix with lemon and orange juice if desired. Stir and serve.

The Big C Fighter

This combination of fruits and vegetables are rich in phytochemicals known to fight carcinogens which may cause cancer. A good source of vitamins, minerals and dietary fiber as well which helps to improve general health.

2 stalks broccoli

½ head of cabbage

½ head of cauliflower

50g spinach

½ lime

3 peaches

Core the peaches and cut a lime in half. Prepare the cabbage and cauliflower. Juice the broccoli, cabbage, cauliflower, spinach, lime and peaches together and serve.

Very Berry Power

Berries contain phytochemicals and flavonoids that may reduce the risk of getting cancer. Blackberries and blueberries specifically are rich in minerals that may prevent bladder infections. This juice mix is a low-calorie source of vitamins and anti-oxidants.

1 cup blackberries

2cups blueberries

2 apples, cored and sliced

Process the fruits in a juicer and serve.

Berry Akai Delight

The acai berry is loaded with phytochemicals known to reduce the risk of cancer, cardiovascular illness and lessen the severity of common ailments such as colds and flu.

½ cup acai berries

½ lemon

½ papaya (peeled)

1 ½ tablespoon honey

Put them all in a juicer and enjoy!

Super Anti-oxidant

Raspberry is a super fruit packed with anti-oxidants, vitamins C, minerals and fibers. The combination of spinach, peach, lime and cucumber make this concoction a super anti-oxidant.

1 cup raspberry

1 ½ cup spinach

1 peach

½ lime

1/2 cucumber

Wash all the ingredients. Run them through a juicer. Take the expelled pulp and run it back through the juicer a second time to extract all liquid. Serve and drink.

Super Colon Cleanser

This juice is loaded with phytochemicals and nutrients as well as dietary fibers that are good for colon and gallbladder cleansing.

2 apples

½ medium carrots

4 slices of medium cucumber

2 stalks of celery

½ tbsp of honey

Mix the apple, celery, carrot, cucumber, lemon juice and honey in your juicer. Puree into a shake. Drink immediately before it oxidizes.

Cholesterol Fighter

This nutritious drink is low in cholesterol but rich in anti-oxidants, vitamins, minerals and dietary fiber which helps control blood cholesterol levels, prevents constipation, protects body from free radicals mediated injury and from cancers.

5 carrots

7 stalks celery with leaves

8 stems parsley with leaves

3 garlic cloves

Juice all the ingredients together and you're done. Stir and serve.

Cleansing Veggie Combi

Rich in vitamins and minerals, vegetables are also a good source of dietary fiber which is a natural body cleanser. This combination of vegetables is ideal for a weight loss regimen since they are all low in calories.

2 cups kale leaves
2 stalks celery
1cup beets
1 turnip
½ cup spinach
½ head bok choy
2 cups parsley
2 garlic cloves

Juice all ingredients in a juicer until smooth. Drink up and enjoy!

Liver Cleansing Juice Drink

Over exposure to toxins may over-stress the liver and affect the other organs resulting to common symptoms such as headaches, muscle pain, fatigue, poor coordination, nerve problems, skin irritations and emotional imbalances. This juice can help cleanse the liver from harmful toxins. Loaded with anti-oxidant compounds, it can also help boost immune system and protect the body against cancer.

2 cups grape
5 stalks chard
1 grapefruit
½ lime

Process all ingredients in a juicer. Stir and enjoy!

Fiery Fruity Drink

Chili peppers have amazingly high levels of vitamins

and minerals. They specifically contain capsaicin which has anti-bacterial, anti-carcinogenic, analgesic and anti-diabetic properties. They also help reduce the cholesterol levels in the blood.

2 whole green peppers
2 ¼ tbsps of honey
½ lime
1 apple

Clean the chili peppers and remove the seeds. Peel the lime and wash the apple. Mix the apple, chili peppers and lime in the juicer. Then add the honey into the finished juice until it fully dissolves. Stir and drink.

Everyday Energizer

Low in calories but a good source of energy boosting vitamins, this juice drink is recommended to prevent cancer and booster immunity. Also high in fiber, including the soluble type that lowers elevated blood cholesterol levels.

4 carrots

5 stalks celery

1 cup of parsley

1 cup squash, zucchini

1 small beet chopped

½ inch ginger

½ lemons peeled

Push all ingredients through the juicer and drink up!

Juice Detox

This delicious fruit mix is loaded with vitamins and minerals to cleanse the body and remove toxins and free radicals.

2 cups grapes

2-3 cups strawberries

3 apricots

3 sprigs fresh mint

Combine all ingredients together in the juicer.   Stir and serve.

Skin Cleanser

If you are suffering from skin break-outs, this juice mix can help clear your skin. Cucumber has a cooling and hydrating effect on the skin and combined with the other vegetables which are rich in vitamins and anti-oxidants, your skin will surely benefit from this mix.

1 ½ cucumber with skin
1 cup fresh parsley
½ cup chopped alfalfa sprouts
4 sprigs fresh mint

Combine all ingredients together in the juicer.   Stir and serve.

Sweet and Tangy Drink

This juice recipe combines the taste of earthy vegetables and sweetness of fruits with tangy kale. Rich in anti-oxidants and high in fiber, this is a nutrient-packed drink for the health conscious.

8 medium carrots

2 cups kale leaves

1½ cup turnip

1½ cup parsnip

7 stalks celery

1 rutabaga

¼ head red cabbage.

6 radishes

1 apple

1 cup cranberry

Process the ingredients one by one in a juicer. Combine and enjoy!

The Milk Alternative

Broccoli and kale are excellent sources of calcium and Vitamin K needed for bone health. Along with carrots and apple, this mix is an excellent source of anti-oxidants, vitamins and dietary fiber. As a milk alternative, this is even better than milk.

1 cup broccoli florets

2-3 kale leaves

3-4 medium-sized carrots

Half slice of an apple

Wash carrots thoroughly and remove tops. Put all ingredients together in the juicer, stir and chill.

Fruity Berry

Berries are loaded with antioxidants that help to prevent cancer. They are also loaded with vitamins and minerals to help strengthen arteries and protect them from oxidative damage.

3 cups of strawberries

3 cups of blueberries

1½ cup of choke berry

Wash thoroughly and juice. Drink and enjoy!

Carrot and Ginger Cleanser

Carrots are good sources of beta-carotene, an anti-oxidant and immune booster. This juice blend is rich in dietary fiber, a natural internal body cleanser.

3 cups carrots

½ inch of fresh ginger root

1 orange

Peel the ginger root and carrot before placing them in the juicer. Stir the juice. Serve cold with slices of orange and drink!

Alkaline Juice

Over-acidity in the body tissues can cause arthritic and rheumatic diseases. Symptoms of over-acidity include insomnia, water retention, migraines, and fatigue. Eating alkalizing fruits and vegetables can effectively relieve these symptoms.

1 cucumber peeled

3 stalks of celery

1 ½ large handfuls of turnip greens

3 cloves of garlic peeled

½ lemons peeled

Push all through the juicer. Juice the greens by pushing them down with the cucumber or celery.

Banana Almonds Smoothie

This is a delicious energy-booster drink rich in dietary fiber, vitamins, minerals and packed with numerous health promoting phytochemicals that ensure protection against diseases and cancers.

1cup plum

2 small bananas

1 ½ cup fresh rhubarb

1 ½ tsp. of honey

Process all ingredients in a juicer until smooth. Drink and enjoy!

Blood Pressure Regulator

This is a recipe loaded with anti-oxidants, vitamin C and dietary fiber. This juice can help regulate blood pressure and lower cholesterol as well.

4-5 stalks fresh bokchoy

4-5 stalks of celery

1 ½   cucumber

2 cups fresh spinach leaves

2 ½   apples

Wash vegetables and fruit. Cut all except spinach into smaller pieces to fit into juicer. Put all through juicer. Spinach leaves may be wrapped around the veggies or rolled up to make them easier to juice. Stir and serve.

Bone Strengthener Detox

This is a low calorie juice drink which can help strengthen the bones, and loaded with anti-oxidants to help fight certain kinds of cancer as well. Great for body detox.

1 ½ heads cauliflower

2 cups butternut squash cut into desired size

1/2 lemon

1 apple

2 cups spinach

3 stalks celery with tops

¼ cup romaine lettuce

1 bulb fennel

½ cube ginger

2 cloves garlic

Wash all veggies and run them through the juicer. Run the pulp back through the juicer a second time. Serve and enjoy.

Applelicious Veggie Drink

Apples are low in calories but contain good quantities of vitamin-C and beta-carotene which is a powerful natural antioxidant and helps the body develop resistance against infectious diseases. Vegetables are also loaded with antioxidants that protect the body from oxidant stress and cancers, as well as help boost the immune system.

2 ripe apples

½ cup spinach

1 cup parsley

3 stalks celery

7 stalks napa cabbage

Wash the ingredients and cut into small sections if needed. Juice the apples and set aside. Juice all the remaining ingredients. Add the apples, stir and enjoy.

Pumpkin Power Drink

Pumpkin, by itself, is a storehouse of anti-oxidant vitamins such as A, C and E that helps the body develops resistance against infectious agents and protects it against lung and oral cavity cancers. Added with apple and carrots, this juice combination is a powerhouse of anti-oxidants which also gives protection against damage from free radicals that causes premature ageing.

3 cups pumpkin chunks

2 loquat

3 carrots

1 inch piece ginger

cinnamon

small amount of nutmeg

Cut the pumpkin in half and scoop out the seeds. Cut into 1 1/2 inch chunks and remove skin with a vegetable peeler. Wash apple and carrots and cut into pieces that will fit into your juicer. Put the first four ingredients through your juicer. Pour the juice into a glass and sprinkle with cinnamon and nutmeg. Add ice if desired.

Makes approximately 12 oz.

Green Delight

This juice blend is a good source of anti-oxidants and dietary fiber for protection against certain types of cancer. Drinking this juice regularly helps prevent osteoporosis, relieve constipation and helps the body develop resistance against infectious diseases.

1 apple

2 cucumbers

½ green cabbage

2 cups spinach

Wash fruits and vegetables. Cut to the size that will fit into your juicer. Push the raw foods through the juicer machine. Add ice and enjoy.

Makes approximately10 oz of juice.

The Colors of Summer

The combination of cantaloupe, apple and pineapple makes for a low-calorie drink loaded with anti-oxidant vitamins A and C. These are essential for vision, immunity, healthy mucus membranes and skin. Consumption of natural fruits rich in vitamin-A is known to protect from lung and oral cavity cancers.

Rich in electrolytes and water content, this is an ideal nutritious drink to beat the summer thirst.

½ medium cantaloupes
2 medium apples
½ cup pineapple

Juice ingredients in a juicer until smooth. Drink and enjoy!

Three C's Plus One Juice Drink

This juice is low in calories and rich in vitamins, minerals and anti-oxidants that boost immune system. Drinking this mix can help lower homocysteine levels in the blood, high levels of which can result in the development of coronary heart disease, stroke and peripheral vascular diseases. The vitamin K specifically found in celery also helps strengthen bones.

2 carrots

½ cup chard

3 sticks celery

2 cucumbers

Wash the stuff, cut into small sections if needed. Juice everything together until desired consistency. Stir and enjoy.

Green Cocktail

This juice blend is a storehouse of phytonutrients that promote good health and disease prevention properties. Loaded with vitamins A, B-complex, E and K as well as essential minerals to protect the skin from premature aging and boost the immune system, this green cocktail is ideal for the health-conscious.

2 kale leaves

2 cups spinach

½ peach

½ fresh avocados

½ tbsp flax seed

2 cups green grapes

Process all ingredients in a juicer until smooth. Drink and enjoy!

Spicy Veggie Drink

This juice blend contains no cholesterol but rich in anti-oxidants, vitamins, minerals, dietary fiber and other healthful substances which helps control blood cholesterol levels, prevents constipation, and protects the body against certain cancers.

1 bunch parsley

6 turnips

4 tomatoes

2 red bell peppers

2 onions

1 clove garlic

Wash and Combine all ingredients together in the juicer. Stir, enjoy and relax.

Fresh Vital Green Drink

Kale leaves contain more iron and calcium than most vegetable. Its high vitamin C- content enhances the body to absorb these minerals. This juice blend is also an excellent low-calorie source of lycopene, and anti-oxidant vitamins, minerals as well as dietary fiber that helps to control blood cholesterol levels, and helps fight the cancer-causing chemicals in our body.

3 cups kale leaf
3 cups collard leaf
3 cups parsley
½ green peppers
2 green tomatoes
1 floret broccoli

Wash then combine all ingredients together in the juicer.

Stir and enjoy.

Armor Shield Drink

This juice combination is good source of dietary fiber, beta carotene, folate, vitamin A & C , calcium, potassium and iron that may protect against some intestinal upsets and may help prevent some urinary tract infections, prevent night blindness, ease arthritis pain and help reduce the risk of certain cancers. Try this juice combination in your fasting diet today.

1 cup blueberries

5 medium carrots

2 medium cucumbers

5 celery stalks

2cups beet

1 cup pineapple

Wash all the ingredients, peel the carrots and cucumbers. Combine all ingredients together in the juicer. Stir and serve.

Orangey Avocado Drink

This juice rich in numerous anti-oxidant polyphenolic flavonoids and contains essential fatty acids which are good for your heart and help reduce bad cholesterol. In addition to this, the avocado supplies you with a large quantity of fibers which are good for your digestion. Also, the orange and melon contain a high amount of vitamin C, which help strengthen the immune system.

1 avocado

1 melon

1 orange

4 stalks of fresh cilantro

Combine all ingredients in a juicer. Process and mix well. Add ice cubes, serve cold and enjoy.

Popeye Juice

This vegetable juice combination contains health-promoting phytochemicals that helps protect the body against certain kinds of cancer. It is a very excellent source of vitamin A, C, K, calcium, iron, potassium, and anti-oxidants which are important as intracellular electrolyte, strengthening bone formation, immune system booster, blood pressure reducer and essential for red blood cell formation.

2 cups spinach

2 stalks kale

2 fennel bulbs

2 cups parsley

1 cucumber

1 one-inch cube of ginger

Wash all ingredients. Run them through a juicer. Any pulp should be run through the juicer a second time to extract all juice from the vegetables. Serve and drink.

serve.

Orangey Avocado Drink

This juice rich in numerous anti-oxidant polyphenolic flavonoids and contains essential fatty acids which are good for your heart and help reduce bad cholesterol. In addition to this, the avocado supplies you with a large quantity of fibers which are good for your digestion. Also, the orange and melon contain a high amount of vitamin C, which help strengthen the immune system.

1 avocado
1 melon
1 orange
4 stalks of fresh cilantro

Combine all ingredients in a juicer. Process and mix well. Add ice cubes, serve cold and enjoy.

Popeye Juice

This vegetable juice combination contains health-promoting phytochemicals that helps protect the body against certain kinds of cancer. It is a very excellent source of vitamin A, C, K, calcium, iron, potassium, and anti-oxidants which are important as intracellular electrolyte, strengthening bone formation, immune system booster, blood pressure reducer and essential for red blood cell formation.

2 cups spinach

2 stalks kale

2 fennel bulbs

2 cups parsley

1 cucumber

1 one-inch cube of ginger

Wash all ingredients. Run them through a juicer. Any pulp should be run through the juicer a second time to extract all juice from the vegetables. Serve and drink.

Yummy Green Drink

Spinach is one of the vegetables recommended in cholesterol control and weight reduction. This vegetable and fruit juice combination is a very rich source of heart healthy electrolytes, antioxidant, vitamins and minerals that gives the body energy and immunity resistance against infectious diseases.

1 cup spinach

2 cups kale leaves

1 orange

2 banana

1 kiwi

Wash all ingredients thoroughly. Put all ingredients together in the juicer, stir and drink.

Heart-Friendly Juice

This delicious and refreshing juice drink is full of

anti-oxidants which keep the bad cholesterol away, as well as buffer the effects of free radical damage to the cells caused by oxidation. Pomegranate seeds keep blood platelets from sticking together and forming dangerous blood clots and also increase oxygen levels to the heart. Mango is a very rich source of potassium that helps control heart rate and blood pressure.

2 pomegranates
½ mangos
1 stalk mint

Peel the pomegranate and remove the seeds. Peel the mango, and put both mango and pomegranate in the juice press. Pour the juice in a large glass and add the mint and pomegranate seeds on top. Drink and enjoy.

Tropical Juice Drink

The papain in papaya, bromelain in pineapple, pectin in

orange, astringent properties of guava and the polyphenolic anti-oxidant compounds in mango combine to make this the ultimate juice drink. Rich in essential vitamins and minerals as well as anti-oxidant compounds and dietary fiber, this juice is good for the heart and digestion, has anti-ageing properties, immune booster and anti-cancer, all in one.

2 mangoes
1 large orange
½ pineapple
½ big papaya
1 big guava

Combine all ingredients in the juicer. Stir and enjoy this delicious juice drink.

Berry Guava Mix

Berries contain phytochemicals and flavonoids that may help to prevent some forms of cancer. They are low in calories but rich in vitamins A and C. Guava is also rich in vitamin C as well as dietary fiber to help cleanse the colon.

1 ½ cup strawberry

1 ½ cup raspberries

1 ½ cup blackberries

½ big guava

Process ingredients in the juicer, drink and enjoy!

Asian Flavor Drink

This fruit combination is rich in anti-oxidant vitamins A, C and E, as well as flavonoids such as pectin, a soluble fiber that helps lower cholesterol and blood pressure.

2 pieces kumquat

1 piece tangerine

3 pieces pears

3 pieces apples

Wash all ingredients and run them through the juicer. Stir, serve and enjoy this flavorful drink.

Chlorophyll Juice

Consuming chlorophyll from this juice is a highly effective way to alkalize the blood and energize the body. This juice is a great source of vitamins A, B, C, E, potassium, lutein and carotene which are highly effective in eliminating free radicals and prevent cancer of the lung and prostate. This juice combination has the ability to cleanse the blood, organs and gastrointestinal tract as well as help prevent blindness and lower blood cholesterol levels.

2 cups spinach
1 bunch wheat grass
6 carrots
1 stalk celery

Wash all ingredients and run them through the juicer. Run the pulp back through the juicer a second time. Drink and enjoy.

Tangy Berry Drink

This juice combination is loaded with vitamin C and bioflavonoids that help strengthen immune resistance, lower blood cholesterol and protect against cancer. Add this juice recipe in your diet fasting.

2 tangerines
1 cup raspberry
½ lemon
1 inch ginger

Wash all ingredients and run them through the juicer. Stir, serve and enjoy.

Carroty Green Drink

Juice fasting does no harm and may at the same time confer major health benefits against two leading killers, cancer and heart disease. This juice blend is excellent source of beta carotene, dietary fiber, calcium, iron, potassium, vitamin A and C that help prevent night blindness, protect against cell damage by free radicals, reduce blood sugar levels in diabetics and help heal peptic ulcers.

6 medium carrots
1 bunch watercress
3 cups parsley
1 cup green cabbage

Wash all the ingredients thoroughly. Scrub the carrots and push them through the machine with the watercress leaves, parsley and its stalks and the cabbage. Drink immediately.

Spicy Fiber Drink

This nutritious juice for the weight-conscious is an excellent source of beta carotene and vitamins A, C and E, folate, calcium, and potassium as well as dietary fiber. This juice blend helps alleviate viral infections by boosting immunity. It also helps remove harmful free radicals from the body and protects it from certain kinds of cancer.

2 cups kale
3 apples
3 horseradish
½ lemon
1 stalk celery
½ inch ginger

Wash all ingredients and run them through the juicer. Stir, serve and enjoy.

Refreshing Fruit Drink

An excellent source of vitamin A, C, beta carotene, folate, thiamine and potassium a nutrient essential for healthy hair, skin, eyes, bones, and mucous membranes, this refreshing juice has a menthol taste and a cooling sensation that helps reduce blood cholesterol and blood pressure level.

1 orange

3 carrots

½ papayas

3 apples

1 guava

½ cup peppermint

Wash all ingredients and run them through the juicer. Stir, serve and enjoy.

Veggie Squeeze

This juice blend is an excellent source of antioxidant vitamins A and C as well as potassium that help prevents infections in the body and essential to the diet because they protect against cancer. Try this juice in your fasting diet for effective result.

5 carrots

2 cucumbers

3 stalks celery

2 asparagus

2 zucchinis

Wash all ingredients and combine together in the juicer. Stir and enjoy.

Sunshiny Drink

This juice combination is high in vitamin C and provides a good amount of pectin, a soluble dietary fiber that helps control blood cholesterol levels and boosts the immune system against diseases.

½ orange

2 grapefruit

¼ medium papayas

1 inch ginger

Wash all ingredients and run them through the juicer. Stir, serve and enjoy.

Garden Delight

Collard greens are excellent source of vitamin-A and flavonoids that help improves healthy mucous membranes and skin, also essential for vision. This vegetable juice contains excellent amount of beta carotene, lycopene, folate, vitamin C, calcium, iron, potassium and antioxidants to prevent cancer-causing cell damage, control heart rate, reduce blood pressure, essential for body metabolism and blood cell formation.

4 stalks collard greens

2 cups romaine lettuce leaves

2 skinny carrots

1 cup cauliflower

1 large eggplant

2 stalks celery

3 small peppers

1 medium tomato

Add fresh ground black pepper to taste. Wash all ingredients and run them through the juicer. Stir, serve and enjoy.

Salad Drink

This juice blend is loaded with dietary fiber and vitamins A and C, folate, potassium and lycopene which helps increase bulk of the food by absorbing water throughout the digestive system and helps in easing constipation, treat gout, high blood pressure and protect against some cancers.

1 bunch coriander leaves

4 medium tomatoes

4 stalks celery

1 onion

3 green peppers

Wash all ingredients thoroughly. Put together in the juicer, stir and drink.

Rainbow Drink

This juice is a store house of phytonutrients that have health promotional and disease prevention properties. Loaded with vitamins A, B-complex, C, E, K, pyridoxine, carotenes, omega-fatty acids, riboflavin, and thiamine, this fruit blend helps to protect the body from harmful free radicals and boost the immune system, as well as being anti-inflammatory, anti-ulcer, and anti-cancer.

2 cups kale

2 cups spinach

2 cups lychee

½ fresh avocados

1 cup grapes

2 tbsp hemp seeds

Process all ingredients in a juicer until smooth. Drink and enjoy!

Flavonoid Drink

This juice blend is rich in fiber and flavonoids that helps lower body cholesterol level and improves blood flow. This is also an excellent source of anti-oxidant vitamins A, C and E as well as B-complex and beta carotene that boosts the immune system and protects the body against harmful free radicals.

2 kiwi fruits

2 star fruits

1 medium eggplant

1 medium cucumber

Wash all ingredients and run them through the juicer. Stir, serve and enjoy.

Juicy Greens

Celery, chard and kale are good sources of potassium, folate, calcium, omega-3 fatty acids and bioflavonoids that help protect against certain cancers, retain the elasticity of the arteries, as well as help improve the digestive system and lower cholesterol levels.

3 stalks celery

1 cup green Swiss chard leaf

5 kale leaves

½ pomelo

1 apple

¼ inch ginger

Push all ingredients through the juicer. Juice the greens by pushing them down with fruits. Stir and enjoy.

Leafy Delight

This juice combination is a low-calorie source of dietary fiber that helps reduce weight while preventing constipation and colon-rectal cancer risks; decrease bad cholesterol levels and regulates blood sugar levels. This juice mix is full of antioxidant vitamin A, C, K and B-complex to protect the body against cancer, promote healthy mucus membranes and bone development as well as help the body develop resistance against infectious agents.

1 bunch asparagus
1 handful collard greens
2 stalks celery
1 carrot
1 apple

Wash all ingredients and run them through the juicer. Run the pulp back through the juicer a second time. Serve and enjoy.

Grapefruit Power Juice

Grapefruit contains salicylic acid that helps break down the body's inorganic calcium, which builds up in the cartilage of joints and may lead to arthritis. Sweet potatoes are high in vitamin B6 which helps prevent degenerative diseases including the heart attacks. Peaches are rich in dietary fiber and potassium which acts as a kidney cleanser. All three contain anti-oxidant vitamins and minerals which boost the immune system and fight harmful free radicals.

3 grapefruits
2 sweet potatoes
2 peaches

Process the ingredients in a juicer and serve.

Starry Starry Mix

This vegetable and fruit juice combination contains health-promoting phytochemicals that help protect the body against certain kinds of diseases, especially the antioxidants and bioflavonoids that help block cancer causing substances. This juice is rich in ascorbic acid and bromelain, which is important to keep bones, teeth, mucous membranes, skin and immune system healthy. It also helps to reduce digestive upsets and reduce inflammation. Get your juicer now! Be healthy, be happy.

3 cups spinach

1 ½ star fruit

½ cup pineapples

3 medium cucumbers peeled

Wash all the ingredients. Run them through a juicer. Take the expelled pulp and run it back through the juicer a second time to extract all liquid. Stir and enjoy!

Sweet Melon Mint

This juice combination is a rich source of anti-oxidants such as vitamin C, beta-carotene and lutein which acts as protective scavengers against harmful free radicals that play a role in aging and various disease processes, and potassium which helps reduce blood pressure and heart rates by countering the effects of sodium.

½ honeydew melon

2 medium cucumbers

1 cup mint leaves

1 cup pineapple

3 medium eggplant peeled

Wash then combine all ingredients together in the juicer. Stir and enjoy.

Raisin Alert Mix

This juice combination is ideal for those suffering from high blood pressure, constipation problems, stress, obesity and a lot more. It helps to flush toxins inside the body; helps enhance the immune system and provide essential nutrients and anti-oxidants.

5 apples
3 carrots
½ cup raisins
2 tbsp honey

Wash all the ingredients thoroughly. Scrub the carrots and push them all through the machine. Drink immediately and relax.

Sweet Savory Juice

This juice combination is an excellent source of beta carotene, lycopene, vitamin A, C and potassium which helps lower blood cholesterol levels and prevents certain cancer.

3 pieces large bell pepper

7 carrots

2 medium tomatoes

1 tbsp honey

Wash all ingredients except honey and run them through the juicer. Add honey and stir. Serve and enjoy.

Spare of Asparagus

This juice combination has the highest nutritional value especially for those people suffering from insomnia, irritable bowel syndrome, and blurred vision. This juice blend is also rich in potassium, copper and iron which are important components of cell and body fluids that helps control heart rate, blood pressure, cellular respiration and red blood cell formation.

5 asparagus

2 medium carrots

1 lemon

2 tomatoes

1 tbsp honey

Juice them all and serve!

Sweet Humid Drink

This juice blend is rich in dietary fiber that helps to protect the colon and mucous membrane, helps control heart rate and lower blood pressure. It is an excellent source of vitamins A and C, as well as potassium and beta carotene that help lower blood cholesterol levels, protect against cancer and prevent blindness.

2 cups ripe jackfruit bulbs

3 medium carrots

5 cups spinach

3 stalks celery

2 lemons

½ inch ginger

Wash all ingredients and run them through the juicer. Stir and Enjoy!!

Peach Berry Cocktail

This juice combination provides some vitamin C, iron, potassium, beta carotene, folate and thiamine. It is high in fiber especially pectin, a soluble fiber that is instrumental in lowering high blood cholesterol.

3 peaches

2 orange

1cup blueberries

1 cup cherries

Push fruits through the juicer. Stir, serve and enjoy!

Disease Fighting Juice

This juice blend helps fight heart diseases, diabetes, constipation, cancer, arthritis and high blood pressure. It is rich in antioxidants, omega-3 essential fatty acids, vitamins A, C and K and other essential nutrients.

2 small bananas

1 cup spinach

½ tbsp ground flaxseed

½ tbsp chia seeds

1 apple

Put in the juicer. Process and serve.

Sweet Freshener Juice Drink

Spinach is a rich source of vitamin A and lutein which keeps the eyes and mucous membranes. This juice is abundant with beta carotene, vitamins A, C, E, K, folate, potassium and lycopene that help reduce the risk of macular degeneration, reduce inflammation and protect against cancer. Try this juice with its sweet and menthol taste which is good to relieve, asthma, fatigue and stress.

1 cup spinach

1 medium carrots

1 cup parsley

2 stalks celery

3 medium bell peppers

3 medium tomatoes

½ cup mint leaves

1 tbsp honey

Push all through juicer. Note: mint leaves can be rolled up into a ball to create volume when pushing through the juice extractor. Makes 12 oz of juice. Stir and enjoy!

Jalapeño Madness

Jalapeno pepper has a chemical compound called capsaicin which helps lower blood cholesterol, promotes weight loss and fights against some types of colon and stomach cancers.

2 jalapeno peppers
2 large green peppers
1 cup cilantro
2 green onions
3 large tomatoes
½ avocado

Wash all the ingredients. Run them through a juicer. Take the expelled pulp and run it back through the juicer a second time to extract all liquid. Drink and enjoy!

Green Vapors

The combination of spinach, lettuce, celery, carrots,

cucumbers and a squeeze of lime is effective in body cleansing. Juice is better chilled as possible in the morning before living for work. Keep it cool to help minimize oxidation.

2 cups spinach
2 cups romaine lettuce
2 stalks celery
5 medium carrots
3 medium cucumbers
½ lime

Wash all the ingredients. Run them through a juicer. Take the expelled pulp and run it back through the juicer a second time to extract all liquid. Makes approximately 16 oz of juice. Stir and enjoy!

Body Toxin Cleanser

Dietary cholesterol is the type consumed in foods specifically animal products and junk foods. The body does not need this cholesterol; they can cause certain diseases. To wash out this type of toxin inside the body, try this juice combination. It is recommended as an effective body toxin cleanser.

1 medium apple

2 cups spinach

2 cups parsley

2 large carrots

1 cup celery r leaves

1 medium beet root with green tops

Wash all the ingredients. Run them through a juicer. Take the expelled pulp and run it back through the juicer a second time to extract all liquid. Stir the juice and serve immediately for the greatest nutritional benefits.

Pea and Basil Juice

Besides being high in protein, fresh green peas are good

sources of pectin and other soluble fiber, which help control blood cholesterol levels. This juice mix is full of digestion friendly fiber to help prevent cardiovascular disease and constipation. It also contains many polyphenolic flavonoids known to have anti-inflammatory and anti-bacterial properties as well as high amount of iron which is very important in the production of healthy red blood cells.

1 cup sweet peas
3 stalks celery with leaves
1 tomato
½ garlic clove
5 cups basil leaves

Rinse the vegetables first and then put the peas, celery leaves and tomatoes into the juicer. Squeeze garlic with basil in a different container. Pour the juice into a glass, and mix in the garlic-basil. Stir and serve.

Pepper Bell

Fresh red and green peppers are rich sources of vitamin C which is a potent water soluble antioxidant. It is required for the collagen synthesis in the body in maintaining the integrity of blood vessels, skin, organs, and bones. This juice is loaded with vitamins, minerals and antioxidants. This juice is good source of dietary fiber that helps reduce constipation, promote weight loss, helps control heart rate and blood pressure.

1green peppers
1 red pepper
2celery stalks
1cucumber
2 cups lettuce leaves

Wash thoroughly and combine all ingredients in the juicer. Stir and serve.

Fruitgrass Combi

More than ever, people are realizing that what they eat does make a difference, not only in the way they look and feel but also in the length and quality of their lives. To obtain a healthy body, follow a healthy and balance diet. Try this juice combination for an effective body detoxification.

1 cup grapes
½ cup pineapple
½ cup wheat grass

Juice all the ingredients together and you're done. Stir and serve.

Orange Wheat

Try this juice with wheatgrass combination to help the body fight against common diseases and certain kinds of cancer. This combination is rich in antioxidant vitamins A, C and E which are important for immune function to ward off infection and strengthening the blood vessel walls.

2 bunch wheatgrass

1 inch piece fresh ginger

5 pieces oranges

Wash all the ingredients. Run them through a juicer. Take the expelled pulp and run it back through the juicer a second time to extract all liquid. Stir juice and serve immediately for the greatest nutritional benefit.

Tomato Desire

This juice blend is an excellent low calorie source of vitamins A, C, potassium and lycopene. It can help lower the risk of prostate cancer in men and reduce inflammation. It also helps lower blood pressure and cholesterol levels.

3 ripe tomatoes

2 green peppers

2 stalks celery

2 apples

2 onions

Wash all ingredients and run them through the juicer. Run the pulp back through the juicer a second time. Serve and enjoy.

Walnut Harmony

Research shows that consumption of small amounts of walnuts is linked to decreased risk of heart disease, certain kinds of cancer, gallstones, type 2 diabetes and other health problems. This juice combination is rich in anti-oxidants which protect the body against the damaging effects of free radicals and other food chemicals.

4 apples

2 stalks celery with leaves

1 cup grapes

1 cup walnuts

Wash all ingredients thoroughly. Put all ingredients together in the juicer, stir and drink.

Alpha Mix

Juice fasting is highly recommended to relieve symptoms, maintain good health and promote healing, not to replace the medicines and surgery that doctors use to treat illness but to help them prevent the risk of the disease and help the immune system to fight illnesses. This juice blend is a storehouse of phytonutrients that promote good health and disease prevention properties.

2 medium sweet potatoes peeled

2 orange

2 red capsicum

2 red beets root

2 apples

Wash all ingredients and run them through the juicer. Run the pulp back through the juicer a second time. Serve and enjoy.

Colorful Green Juice

This juice combination is loaded with vitamins A and C, calcium, lycopene, iron and potassium that are essential cancer fighting agents. It also prevents night blindness, helps lower blood cholesterol levels and helps reduce inflammation.

3 cups spinach
3 cups romaine leaves
1 medium tomato
2 medium cucumber peeled
2 medium skinny carrots
2 medium radish
2 stalks celery

Add fresh ground black pepper to taste. Wash all ingredients and run them through the juicer. Stir, serve and enjoy.

Blood Booster

This juice combination contains bioflavonoids; plant pigments that may help prevent or retard tumor growth. This is an excellent source of essential nutrients which help control blood cholesterol levels, promotes normal bowel function and also reduce the action of platelets, the blood cells that are instrumental in forming clots.

2 oranges

3 pears

2 yams

2 cups grapes

2 apples

Wash all ingredients and run them through the juicer.

Run the pulp back through the juicer a second time. Serve and enjoy.

Fruity Delight

This juice combination is low in calorie and excellent source of vitamins B, C, beta carotene, folate, thiamine and potassium which help protect against cell damage caused by free radicals produced when oxygen is burned in the human body, as well as help reduce the risk of certain cancers, heart attacks, and strokes.

¼ watermelons

1 lemon

6 oranges

2 cups pineapple

2 bananas

Wash all ingredients and run them through the juicer. Stir, serve and enjoy.

Delightfully Sweet Juice

This sweet smelling juice will give a much needed vitamin and mineral boost without the heavy calories. A good source of thiamin, riboflavin, vitamin A, vitamin C and iron, incorporate this juice in your juice fasting recipe.

1piece cantaloupe chopped
3 pieces sweet potatoes peeled
pinch of cinnamon
2 tbsp. sucanat

Wash cantaloupe and potatoes; process together in the juicer. Add the sucanat and cinnamon. Stir and enjoy.

Olympic Flavor

Coconut meat contains lauric acid which helps fight bacteria from intestinal parasites and wards off countless infections ranging from HIV to the common cold. Coconut water helps the kidney and bladder maintain proper functioning. Spinach and peach are rich in fiber and potassium, as well as beta-carotene, an anti-oxidant that converts to vitamin A which is essential for healthy heart and eyes. Spinach is also loaded with calcium, folic acid, vitamins K, lutein, and iron. Combine these three and you have a nutritious powerhouse.

1-½ cup coconut water
½ cup young coconut meat
2 medium peaches
3 cups fresh spinach

Wash all ingredients and run them through the juicer. Run the pulp back through the juicer a second time. Serve and enjoy.

Optimum Drink

This juice recipe is a low-calorie anti-oxidant packed

drink, ideal for juice fasting. The anti-oxidant vitamins and minerals in this fruit and vegetable combination fight against breast, colon and prostate cancers and help reduce LDL or "bad cholesterol" levels in the blood.

3 apples
2 pieces fresh green Chinese cabbage
½ tbsp. cinnamon
2 tbsp. honey

Wash all the ingredients. Run them through a juicer. Take the expelled pulp and run it back through the juicer a second time to extract all liquid. Stir juice and serve immediately for the greatest nutritional benefit.

Cocoberry Softee

Coconut has many bioactive compounds that are essential for better health. Especially the cytokinins found in coconut water that help slow down the effect of aging, eliminate cancer-causing substances and prevent the formation of blood clot. Try this juice now! It helps build all body tissues, keeps the skin soft and smooth and help lubricates the various organs and joints.

¼ cup young coconut meat

½ cup coconut juice

2 cups blackberries

2 kiwi fruits

½ cup pineapple chopped

¼ pears

Wash all ingredients and run them through the juicer. Run the pulp back through the juicer a second time. Serve and enjoy.

Coco Loco Delight

Coconut, banana and spinach all contain the electrolyte potassium that help maintain fluid balance, promote proper metabolism and muscle function and help maintain proper function of kidney and bladder. The coconut meat contains lauric acid which is beneficial in fighting off infections. This juice provides an excellent amount of calcium, folic acid, vitamins K, lutein, and iron.

1 cup coconut water
1 cup young coconut meat
2large bananas
3 cups fresh spinach

Wash all the ingredients. Run them through a juicer. Take the expelled pulp and run it back through the juicer a second time to extract all liquid. Stir juice and serve immediately for the greatest nutritional benefit.

Tummy Cleaner

This juice blend is an abundant source of anti-oxidants, beta carotene, vitamin C and E. It also contains bioflavonoids and insoluble fiber that protect against cancer and helps regular bowel movement.

3 cups kale leaves

1 large cucumber peeled

1 large green pepper

½ inch ginger

½ tbsp honey

Wash all ingredients and run them through the juicer. Stir, serve and enjoy.

Rootfruity Drink

This juice blend is an excellent source of vitamin C which is necessary to make and maintain collagen, the connective tissue that holds body cells together. It also helps to build teeth and bones, strengthens the walls of capillaries and other blood vessels, as well as promotes healing of wounds and burns. This juice drink also helps the body neutralize carcinogens by protecting its ability to recognize and eliminate malignant cells.

4 carrots peeled

4apples

½ Chinese cabbage

2 turnip roots

Wash all ingredients thoroughly. Put all ingredients together in the juicer, stir and drink.

Vege Warrior

This juice combination is a great source of vitamin C, B6, potassium and other minerals that may protect against cancers and help reduce blood pressure. It also possesses curative power for headaches, gout, inflammatory arthritis, edema and other painful conditions.

2 lemons

2 radishes

1 bunch beet

3 sweet potatoes

3 stalks celery

1 onion

Wash all ingredients and run them through the juicer. Run the pulp back through the juicer a second time. Serve and enjoy.

Veggie Alert

This juice combination is a beneficial source of beta carotene, vitamin C, folate, protein, calcium, iron, potassium. High in fiber, drinking this juice can prevent constipation, night blindness, lower blood cholesterol levels and prevent certain kinds of cancer.

1 head cauliflower

1 head broccoli

7 medium carrots

3 stalks celery

¼ cup fresh dill weed

Wash all the ingredients. Run them through a juicer. Take the expelled pulp and run it back through the juicer a second time to extract all liquid. Makes 20 oz of juice. Stir and enjoy!

Creamy Coco

Coconuts contain lauric acid which has antimicrobial and antibacterial properties. It can help treat asthma, nausea, skin infections, ulcers and other infections. Limiting your diet to juices from fruits and vegetables is a nutritious way to give your digestive system a good rest.

2 cups young coconut meat

1 medium mango, peeled and pitted

½ medium papaya, peeled and pitted

2 tablespoon flax seed

1 maca root

1 head fresh lettuce

Combine all ingredients and run them through the juicer. Stir and serve.

Sweet Yummy

This juice combination is an excellent source of beta carotene, folate, vitamin C, B6 and potassium. Drinking this juice can help ease headaches and other painful conditions, speed up convalescence, lower elevated blood cholesterol, prevent heart attack and protect against cancer. Add this juice in your diet fasting.

2 artichokes
2 yams
2 beets with green tops
1 ½ onion
1lime
½ inch ginger

Wash all ingredients and run them through the juicer.

Stir, serve and enjoy.

Toxic Cleanser

This juice recipe helps protect your liver against damage from toxins. The combination of fruits provide vitamin C, potassium, folate, iron, calcium, bioflavonoids and other plant chemicals that protect against cancer, heart disease and help the body develop resistance against infectious agents. This juice is also rich in vitamin A which helps maintain healthy mucus membranes and prevent skin dryness.

3 apples
½ cup grapefruit
2 cup acai berries
½ lemon
1 handful beet

Juice them all through the juicer. Stir and serve!

Powerful Tonic Drink

This juice blend is an excellent source of vitamin C, beta carotene and flavonoid anti-oxidants. Onion is an effective heart tonic by hindering clot formation. Garlic is a powerful antibiotic and anti-cancer agent. Ginger helps improve the digestion of proteins, protects against the formation of ulcers and reduces intestinal parasites. It is also effective in treating nausea and motion sickness. Combined with astragalus herb, mushroom and broccoli, it can help promote a healthy immune system and prevent cancer.

1 onion diced

8 cloves garlic, minced

1 inch pc fresh ginger, peeled and finely chopped

2 pcs medium carrots

1 slice astragalus root

1 cup fresh mushrooms

1 cup broccoli flowerets

Wash all the ingredients. Run them through a juicer. Take the expelled pulp and run it back through the juicer a second time to extract all liquid. This recipe makes approximately 16 oz of juice. Stir the juice and serve immediately for the greatest nutritional benefit.

Wonder Juice

This juice combination is packed with essential vitamins such as vitamin A, B6, C and thiamine which helps control blood cholesterol levels and prevent some cancers. These nutrients are also essential for healthy hair, skin eyes, bones, and mucous membranes.

1 sweet potato

4 oranges

1 cup strawberry

2 carrots

2 apples

1 papaya

Wash all ingredients and run them through the juicer. Run the pulp back through the juicer a second time.

Serve and enjoy.

Wipe Out Drink

This vegetable mix is a good source of anti-oxidant vitamins A, C, E and K, as well as potassium, manganese, zinc and flavonoids that help block cancer causing substances and bolster immunity. This is an excellent source of beta carotene, a nutrient that is essential for healthy hair, skin, eyes, bones and mucous membranes.

3 cups spinach

2 medium carrots

2 medium beet roots

1 large onion

2 stalks celery

1 cup parsley

2 medium tomatoes

½ lemon

1 tbsp honey

Wash all ingredients and run them through the juicer. Stir, serve and enjoy. This recipe makes 26 oz of juice.

Tasty Tangy Kale

This juice blend contains lycopene and endolse, compounds that can lessen the cancer-causing potential of estrogen and induce production of enzymes that protect against diseases. This juice is a rich source of vitamin A, C, potassium and beta carotene which are beneficial for the heart and help in lowering the cholesterol level.

7 large kale leaves

7 large romaine leaves

2 large stalks celery

4 large carrots

1 inch ginger

2 medium tomatoes

Wash all ingredients and run them through the juicer. Stir, serve and enjoy.

Orange and Avocado Juice

This juice blend is rich in anti-oxidant polyphenolic flavonoids and contains essential fatty acids which are good for the heart and help reduce bad cholesterol. In addition to this, drinking this juice supplies you with dietary fibers which are good for your digestion. Also contains a high amount of vitamin C which helps strengthen the immune system.

1avocado

1 melon

1 orange

4 stalks of fresh cilantro

Add the peeled avocado and cilantro into a blender. Secondly, add peeled melon and orange into the juice press. Mix this with the avocado. Add ice cubes, serve cold and enjoy.

Tropical Sweet Magic

This juice combination is high in fiber and an excellent source of beta carotene, vitamins C, E, potassium and iron. It contains pectin, a soluble fiber that is instrumental in lowering high blood cholesterol. This juice can help protect against some intestinal upsets, and prevent urinary tract infections. Try this sweet and tangy recipe in your juice fasting.

2 peaches
1 cup pineapple
2 mangoes
1 cup blueberries
1 tbsp honey
½ inch ginger

Wash all ingredients and run them through the juicer. Stir, serve and enjoy.

Prime Memory Booster

This drink has a slightly nutty flavor. It is an excellent source of choline, vitamin B and minerals that help increase neurotransmitter acetylcholine substance responsible for improving human memory.

6large carrots
4 stalks celery, with leaves
½ head cabbage
½ lemon

Wash all the ingredients. Run them through a juicer. Take the expelled pulp and run it back through the juicer a second time to extract all liquid. Stir the juice and serve immediately for the greatest nutritional benefit.

Thirsty Mint

This juice is rich in electrolytes and water content that

can beat tropical summer thirst. This juice combination is an excellent source of Vitamin A, C, folate, potassium and iron as well as pectin that help control blood cholesterol levels and essential for vision and immunity. Added mint taste helps relieve fatigue and stress.

¼ watermelon

2 pears

1 lemon

1 handful mint

Wash all ingredients and run them through the juicer. Stir, serve and enjoy.

Green Carroty Juice

This juice combination is rich in antioxidants compounds, minerals and vitamin A, B-complex, and vitamin C. Drinking this juice can help in lowering blood cholesterol level, weight reduction, red blood cell production, anti-aging, constipation relief, sperm production, clear vision, growth development and controlling heart rate.

2 stalks celery with leaves
4 cups spinach
1/3 melon
3 carrots
2 apples

Wash all the ingredients. Run them through a juicer. Take the expelled pulp and run it back through the juicer a second time to extract all liquid. Serve and drink.

Tropical Smoothie

This juice combination is a storehouse of vitamins C and E, beta carotene, folate, niacin, iron and potassium that help prevent cancer as well as treat liver and intestinal disorders. This juice is high in pectin, a soluble fiber that is important in controlling blood cholesterol.

2 orange

1 cup gooseberry

2 mangoes

Process all ingredients in a juicer until smooth. Drink up and enjoy!

CamuCamu Fruit Mix

This juice combination contain no saturated fats but rich in pectin, a dietary fiber that helps lower blood cholesterol levels, decrease the risk of coronary artery disease and heart attacks due to atherosclerosis. Camucamu berries are rich in vitamin C which is needed for the production of strong connective tissues as well as strengthening the immune system.

5 pieces camucamus

3 pieces oranges

1 cup strawberries

production, anti-aging, constipation relief, sperm production, clear vision, growth development and controlling heart rate.

2 stalks celery with leaves
4 cups spinach
1/3 melon
3 carrots
2 apples

Wash all the ingredients. Run them through a juicer. Take the expelled pulp and run it back through the juicer a second time to extract all liquid. Serve and drink.

Tropical Smoothie

This juice combination is a storehouse of vitamins C and E, beta carotene, folate, niacin, iron and potassium that help prevent cancer as well as treat liver and intestinal disorders. This juice is high in pectin, a soluble fiber that is important in controlling blood cholesterol.

2 orange

1 cup gooseberry

2 mangoes

Process all ingredients in a juicer until smooth. Drink up and enjoy!

CamuCamu Fruit Mix

This juice combination contain no saturated fats but rich in pectin, a dietary fiber that helps lower blood cholesterol levels, decrease the risk of coronary artery disease and heart attacks due to atherosclerosis. Camucamu berries are rich in vitamin C which is needed for the production of strong connective tissues as well as strengthening the immune system.

5 pieces camucamus

3 pieces oranges

1 cup strawberries

2 pieces red apples

Wash all the ingredients. Run them through a juicer. Take the expelled pulp and run it back through the juicer a second time to extract all liquid. This recipe makes approximately 16 oz. of juice. Stir juice and serve immediately for the greatest nutritional benefit.

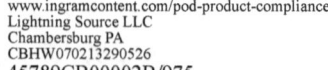